A CODIFICATION OF LONGEVITY

The Key to a Longer and Healthier Life

By

Kurt D. Smith

TABLE OF CONTENTS

INTRODUCTION TO LONGEVITY

The study of longevity in medicine teaches us how to live longer, better lives. Its primary objective is to guarantee that we continue to live healthy, active, and productive lives as we age, in addition to extending our longevity. Living a longer and healthier life is what is meant to be understood as longevity. It indicates a person's expected lifespan and level of health in subsequent years. The state in which an individual lives longer than their average life expectancy is also referred to as longevity.

The term "longevity" describes how long a person has lived, particularly in relation to the population's average lifetime. People from various areas of life are united by the common objective of living a long life, regardless of their background. Building behaviors that will increase your lifespan—such as leading a healthier lifestyle, abstaining from bad habits, getting the care you need, and making educated food choices—is essential to improving your longevity. You can be stated to have durability in case you outlive the standard individual. To stay an extended life, intention to your most ability age. Healthy attitudes and habits can perhaps help achieve this.

The definition of durability is "a high-quality length of life" or "lengthy life. The Latin word longaevitās is where the term originates. This word demonstrates how the terms longus (long) and aevum (age) come together to signify a person who lives a long period of time. This definition's comparison aspect is its most crucial component. The average lifespan is what is meant to be implied by the term "long life.

Longevity is frequently defined by biologists as the typical lifespan anticipated in optimal circumstances. It's difficult to define perfection. There is a lot of current medical research being conducted to determine the "right" kind and quantity of exercise, the optimal diet to follow in order to promote longevity, and whether or not specific medications or supplements can lengthen one's life. Over the past century or so, life expectancy has improved significantly, largely as a result of medical advancements that have almost completely eradicated some fatal infectious diseases. A newborn born in 1900 had a half-century lifespan on average. According to the National Center for Health Statistics, the average life expectancy in the United States today is around 79 years, with 81 years for women and 76 years for men. 2018 mortality in the United States; life expectancy is significantly longer in numerous other countries. The likelihood that humans will live substantially longer in real life is very real. If humans can establish the ideal circumstances of a nutritious diet and regular exercise, they may live longer.

Three ideas are involved in longevity:

1. Prolonging a person's life

2. Improving a person's health (health span; longer life free from illness)

3. managing and reversing aging's telltale signs

Although you may believe that your genes dictate how long you live, genetics actually only determines up to 30% of your life expectancy. The remainder is determined by your actions, mindset, surroundings, and a small amount of good fortune. It's possible that you've heard of several methods for extending life. Remember that none of these have been validated on human subjects, and the majority are merely conjectures. Maintaining good health is the only known way to extend one's life. While there isn't always a perfect way of living, establishing the following behaviors can increase lifespan:

• Engage in physical activity.

• Consume a balanced diet.

• Get seven to 9 hours of sleep each night.

• Practice stress management techniques such as deep breathing, self-care, setting aside time for relaxation, and interacting with others.

• Socialize with loved ones and friends to reduce stress.

• Steer clear of smoking and binge drinking.

CHAPTER ONE

STRATEGIES TO INCREASE YOUR LIFESPAN; WHAT YOU SHOULD DO TO MAXIMIZE YOUR LONGEVITY AND BEAT THE AVERAGE

Below is a list of items to think about:

1. **Get frequent exercise:** According to research, frequent, moderate exercise can actually reverse the effects of aging on your DNA.

2. **Put as many veggies as possible on your dish:** Although there are many differing opinions regarding the optimal diet to lengthen one's life, almost all diets concur that consuming more veggies is a good idea.

3. **Take into consideration intermittent fasting** (there are numerous ways to accomplish this): It has been demonstrated that fasting greatly increases mice's life span and well-being. Research dating back to the 1930s has demonstrated that calorie restriction increases the longevity of test species, including mice. A 2018 study that was published in Cell Metabolism examined 53 non-obese adult humans over two years. The test group followed a 15% calorie restriction. Comparing the test group to

the control group, metabolic measurements revealed that the test group had fewer signs of oxidative stress or damage.

4. **Get adequate rest:** Seven to nine hours of sleep per night is when most individuals feel the best.

5. **Handle your tension with caution:** Stress can encourage bad habits like smoking and overeating, as well as have detrimental consequences for your body.

6. **Foster intimate connections**: It appears that spending time with our loved ones lengthens our lives, perhaps as a result of reducing stress or risky conduct. According to a study conducted by experts at the University of Exeter Medical School in England, the death rate for volunteers was 22% lower than that of non-volunteers.

7. **Give up smoking and heavy alcohol consumption**: Today, resolve to implement one healthy adjustment per week. You'll soon be feeling better and heading toward a long life.

ELEMENTS THAT IMPACT YOUR LONGEVITY

The number of years and quality of your life may depend on several variables. Among these are:

1. **Genetics:** Genetics plays a role in longevity. Research indicates that approximately 25% of the variations in lifespan observed in individuals are attributed to hereditary factors. These gene variants are in charge of protecting the cell against the telltale signs of aging. They are in charge of preserving the ends of chromosomes, fixing DNA, and shielding the cell from oxidative stress, which is caused by mitochondria producing reactive oxygen species

2. **The surroundings**: An individual's environment is a major factor in their longevity. For instance, air quality is one of the environmental elements. Because fewer cars and factories were releasing toxins into the air during the shutdown, fewer people died throughout Europe. Living at higher elevations is another aspect of the environment that can increase lifespan. • You may be surprised to learn that there are a few places on the globe known as "Blue Zones" where people live longer and are less likely to develop chronic illnesses. These Blue Zones are placed in Sardinia, Italy; Okinawa, Japan; Ikaria, Greece; Nicoya, Costa Rica; and Loma Linda, California.

3. **Lifestyle**: Your lifestyle decisions have a direct impact on your health and lifespan, in addition to hereditary and environmental influences. A well-planned physical regimen plus a nutritious diet can improve health and lengthen life. It's crucial to remember that each person is unique, so what works for you might not necessarily work for someone else. To maximize your longevity, it is advisable to base your lifestyle decisions on the findings of your individual medical diagnostics.

CHAPTER TWO

WHICH DIAGNOSTICS EXIST FOR LONGEVITY?

The goal of the Healthy Longevity Clinic is to change the focus of medicine from curing disease to preventing it. Monitoring your body provides information on how to manage aging and encourage a longer, healthier life. For this reason, we always begin each treatment with a thorough, highly customized lifespan diagnosis. To evaluate lifespan, we employ a variety of diagnostic techniques, including physiological measurements, genetic screening, and epigenetic clocks.

Screening by genetics: The goal of genetic screening is to measure your genetic susceptibility to specific diseases. Numerous possible genetic variations that reduce life have been found by scientists. Certain disorders like dementia, cancer, and heart disease may become more likely as a result of these genetic risk variants. In order to reduce negative consequences, individuals with these variations should aspire to a healthy lifestyle from an early age. To find out more, schedule a free appointment with a longevity specialist.

Physiological evaluations: As you age, your cells undergo several changes. A portion of these alterations are microscopic, resulting in cellular abnormalities that have numerous physiological ramifications. The following physiological tests can be used to measure health at a health or longevity clinic today:

• Pulse wave velocity for cardiovascular aging: As people age, their arteries tighten and their heart's capacity to expand decreases. It is recommended to test for an ECG and tonometry (which measures ocular pressure).

• Heart rate variability: As people age, a shift in this variability is eventually linked to heart failure. Therefore, any cardiac aging intervention should show a return to more youthful patterns.

• Grip strength and mortality: Several studies have found a high association between decreased grip strength and mortality. Grip strength is correlated with mortality as well as certain disorders, including frailty in general and cardiovascular issues in particular. In geriatric medicine, it is now considered the "gold standard" and ought to be examined both prior to and following any aging intervention.

• Visceral fat accumulation: Studies have linked visceral fat, particularly in relation to cardiovascular health, to all-cause mortality and increases with age.

• Vital lung capacity (VO2 max): As we age, our ability to exercise is reduced due to a loss in lung function. Both plethysmography and spirometry can be used to quantify it.

The clocks of epigenetics: The epigenome is something you inherit in addition to your parents' genome. Gene expression is regulated by the epigenome through particular mechanisms. The epigenetic areas that regulate age-related illnesses are the focus of epigenetic clocks. The Grim Age clock is now the most accurate predictor of mortality endpoints.

Maintaining a healthy diet and regular exercise can help you live a longer life. A number of other variables, such as binge eating and excessive alcohol consumption, may raise your chance of developing specific illnesses. Many people believe that heredity has a major role in determining life expectancy. Genes, however, are far less important than previously thought. It seems that the important environmental influences are lifestyle and diet. These behaviors are associated with a long life.

There is currently a lot of interest in the relationship between calorie intake and longevity. According to animal research, a typical calorie intake reduction of 10% to 50% may lengthen one's maximum lifetime. Research on human populations known for their long lifespans also shows associations between low calorie intake, a longer life expectancy, and a decreased risk of disease. Additionally, cutting calories may aid in the reduction of excess body weight and abdominal fat, both of which are linked to shortened life spans.

Nevertheless, prolonged calorie restriction is frequently unsustainable and might have unfavorable side effects such as heightened hunger, lowered body warmth, and decreased libido. It's still unclear if cutting calories slows down aging or lengthens life.

Consume more nuts:

Nuts are a powerful source of nourishment. They are abundant in fiber, protein, antioxidants, and healthy plant chemicals. Additionally, they're an excellent source of copper, magnesium, potassium, folate, niacin, and vitamins B6 and E, among other vitamins and minerals. **Nuts are beneficial for heart disease, hypertension, inflammation, diabetes, metabolic syndrome, belly fat, and even some types of cancer, according to several studies.**

According to one study, those who ate three or more servings of nuts a week had a 39% decreased chance of dying young. In a similar vein, two recent assessments involving over 350,000 individuals reported that consuming one serving of nuts weekly reduced the risk of all-cause mortality by 4% and that consuming one serving of nuts daily reduced the risk of CVD mortality by 27%.

OVERVIEW: You might live a longer and healthier life if you include nuts in your daily diet. Try using some turmeric. Turmeric is a fantastic choice for anti-aging tactics. This is because of the presence of curcumin, a strong bioactive ingredient, in this spice. Curcumin is believed to help preserve lung, heart, and brain function as well as guard against cancer and age-related disorders because of its anti-inflammatory and antioxidant qualities. In insects and mice, curcumin has been associated with longer lifespans. Human in vivo and in vitro research has verified that curcumin may aid in the prevention of diabetes, inflammatory diseases, neurodegenerative disorders, cardiovascular diseases, and other ailment. However, turmeric is generally regarded as safe because it has been consumed for thousands of years in India.

The primary bioactive component of turmeric, curcumin, possesses anti-inflammatory and antioxidant properties. According to several studies on animals, it may lengthen life.

Consume a lot of nutritious plant foods:

Eating a diverse range of plant foods, including whole grains, beans, nuts, seeds, fruits, and vegetables, may reduce the risk of disease and lengthen life. A plant-rich diet, for instance, has been associated in numerous studies with a lower risk of cancer, metabolic syndrome, heart disease, depression, and brain degradation, among other conditions. The minerals and antioxidants found in plant diets, such as polyphenols, carotenoids, folate, and vitamin C, are responsible for these effects. Consequently, a number of studies associate diets that are naturally higher in plant foods.

vegetarian and vegan: with a 12–15% decreased risk of dying young. According to the same studies, there is also a 29–52% decreased chance of dying from heart, kidney, or hormone-related disorders, as well as cancer. Furthermore, some studies indicate that consuming more meat may raise the chance of developing certain diseases and dying young. Other studies, however, show either no correlation at all or a significantly weaker one, with processed meat appearing to be particularly associated with negative consequences. Additionally, compared to meat eaters, vegetarians and vegans typically have greater health consciousness, which may help to explain these results. In general, consuming a lot of plant-based foods is probably going to improve longevity and health. Consuming a lot of plant-based foods will probably extend your life and reduce your chance of developing a number of prevalent illnesses.

Continue to exercise:

It should come as no surprise that maintaining an active lifestyle can prolong your life and keep you healthy. You may benefit from exercising for as little as 15 minutes a day, which might add three years to your life. Additionally, for every 15 minutes extra you spend exercising each day, your chance of dying young may drop by 4%. Even though these adults exercised for fewer than the recommended 150 minutes per week, a recent assessment found that those over 60 who exercised had a 22% decreased chance of dying young. Individuals who met the 150-minute recommendation had a 28% lower risk of dying young. Furthermore, 35% of those who exercised in excess of this advice did so. Lastly, studies show that, compared to low- or moderate-intensity activities, vigorous activity reduces risk by 5% more.

OVERVIEW: Engaging in regular physical activity can increase your lifespan. The ideal amount of exercise is above 150 minutes each week, although even small amounts might be beneficial.

Avoid smoking

Smoking has a high correlation with disease and premature mortality. In general, smokers may lose up to ten years of life and have a threefold increased risk of dying young compared to those who never light up. According to a recent assessment, almost all of the elevated risks of death from smoking can be avoided by giving up tobacco use before the age of 40. Remember that you can always give up at any time. According to one study, those who give up smoking before the age of 35 may live an additional 8 years. Moreover, you may add 3 years to your life if you stop smoking in your 60s. Actually, there might still be advantages to stopping in your 80s.

OVERVIEW: It is never too late to stop smoking, and it can greatly extend your life.

Consume alcohol in moderation.

Excessive alcohol intake is associated with an increased risk of premature death overall as well as liver, heart, and pancreatic diseases. On the other hand, moderate intake has been linked to a 17–18% lower risk of dying young and a decreased propensity to get a number of diseases. Because wine contains a lot of polyphenol antioxidants, it is thought to be especially healthy.

Men who favored wine were 34% less likely to die young than those who chose beer or spirits, according to the findings of a 29-year study.

Furthermore, a review found that wine has a particularly strong preventive effect against heart disease, diabetes, neurological conditions, and metabolic syndrome. It is advised that women strive for 1-2 units per day and a maximum of 7 units per week to maintain moderate consumption. Men should consume no more than three units per day and no more than fourteen units per week. It's crucial to remember that there isn't any solid evidence to support the claim that moderate alcohol consumption has more advantages than abstinence. Put another way, if you don't normally drink, there's no need to start now.

OVERVIEW: If you consume alcohol, keeping your consumption in check could help you live a longer and healthier life. Wine could be especially helpful.

Put your happiness first.

Your longevity can be greatly increased by being happy. Over the course of a 5-year study, happy people actually had a 3.7% decrease in premature death. In a study, 180 Catholic nuns' self-reported levels of pleasure upon entering the monastery were examined, and these levels were then compared to the sisters' lifespans. Six decades later, the likelihood of survival for those who were happiest at age 22 was 2.5 times higher.

OVERVIEW: It's conceivable that happiness extends your life and improves your mood. Steer clear of long-term worry and tension. Stress and anxiety can shorten your life expectancy considerably. For example, it has been stated that women who experience stress or anxiety have a twofold increased risk of dying from lung cancer, heart disease, or stroke. Similarly, men who experience anxiety or stress have a three-times higher chance of dying young than men who have a more calm lifestyle. Laughter and optimism can be two important parts of the remedy if you're feeling stressed. According to studies, those who are pessimistic have a 42% higher chance of dying young than those who are more optimistic. But having a cheerful attitude toward life and laughing can both help you feel less stressed, which may help you live a longer life.

Your life expectancy can be increased by learning techniques to manage your stress and worry. Keeping a positive attitude about life might also be helpful.

Take care of your social network

According to research, having strong social networks can increase your chances of surviving by 50%. As a matter of fact, your chances of dying young can be reduced by about 200%

with just three social connections. Additionally, studies have shown that having a healthy social network can improve immunological, hormonal, cardiac, and brain function, all of which can lower your chance of developing chronic illnesses. Strong social ties may also mitigate the detrimental effects of stress, which could account for the longevity benefit. Lastly, a study suggests that helping others may be more advantageous than getting help yourself. Make sure to repay your friends and relatives for their caregiving as well as accept it.

OVERVIEW: Strong connections can lead to lowered stress levels, stronger immunity, and longer life spans.

Exercise greater diligence:

Conscientiousness is the capacity for self-control, efficiency, organization, and goal-setting. Children who were seen as persistent, orderly, and disciplined lived 11% longer than their less conscientious peers, according to data from a study that tracked 1,500 boys and girls into old age. Along with a decreased risk of diabetes, heart disease, and joint issues, conscientious people may also have lower blood pressure and fewer mental health issues. This may be partially due to the fact that conscientious people are more likely to have successful careers or take good care of their health and are less inclined to take risks or react poorly to stress. Even modest actions like keeping a workplace clean, adhering to a schedule, or arriving on time can help someone become more conscientious at any point in life.

OVERVIEW: A longer lifespan and fewer health issues in old age are linked to conscientiousness.

Sip tea or coffee

A lower risk of chronic disease has been associated with both tea and coffee. For example, green tea's polyphenols and catechins may lower your risk of diabetes, heart disease, and cancer. Likewise, coffee consumption is associated with a decreased risk of heart disease, type 2 diabetes, certain malignancies, and neurological conditions including Parkinson's and Alzheimer's. Furthermore, compared to non-drinkers, coffee and tea drinkers enjoy a 20–30% decreased chance of dying young. Just keep in mind that consuming too much caffeine can also cause anxiety and insomnia, so you might want to limit your daily intake to the 400 mg advised, or around 4 cups of coffee. It's also important to remember that the benefits of caffeine usually wear off after six hours. Therefore, you might wish to switch to consuming it earlier in the day if you struggle to obtain adequate restful sleep.

SUMMARY: Drinking tea and coffee in moderation may promote longevity and healthy aging.

Establish a healthy sleeping schedule:

Sleep is essential for controlling how cells function and for physical healing. According to a new study, regular sleeping habits, such as going to bed and waking up at roughly the same time every day, are probably linked to lifespan. Sleep duration appears to be an influence as well, with excessive or insufficient sleep being detrimental. For example, a 12% increased chance of dying young is associated with sleeping fewer than 5–7 hours per night, and a 38% reduction in lifespan is associated with sleeping more than 8–9 hours per night. In addition to increasing inflammation, getting too little sleep can raise your risk of obesity, diabetes, and heart disease. These are all associated with a reduced lifespan. Conversely, sleeping too much may increase your risk of depression, inactivity, and unidentified medical disorders, all of which shorten your life expectancy

OVERVIEW: You could live longer if you establish a sleep schedule that allows you to get 7–8 hours of sleep per night. In summary Even if it seems uncontrollable, a number of healthy behaviors will help you live a long and healthy life. A plant-based diet, stopping smoking, managing stress, exercising, and getting adequate sleep are a few of these. For your long-term health and well-being, you should also limit your alcohol intake, discover joy, drink coffee or tea, and practice conscientiousness. When combined, these practices can improve your health and set you up for a long life.

CHAPTER THREE

RIGHT EATING PATTERN FOR LONGEVITY

A diet with high nutritional content for brain function and health has significant "value for improving cognitive functioning, particularly during aging. Along with bettering brain function, these diets are linked to decreased illness risk and overall wellness, all of which are necessary for a long and healthy life. Good nutrition is essential, but knowing what, how much, and when to eat can be challenging at times. It is even more crucial to monitor the nutrient profile of your diet and make sure it is formulated with nutrition for both brain health and longevity, as nutritional requirements vary with age.

A diet that is longevity-focused prioritizes essential foods and substances that have been scientifically shown to lengthen lifespans. This entails adding the essential nutrients listed below to maintain your health. Antioxidants. Antioxidants function as protectors against the harmful consequences of oxidative stress, a condition linked to aging and cellular damage. According to research, "dietary antioxidants are used in several approaches to improve human health and achieve longevity," including: Vitamin C, Vitamin E Beta-carotene Selenium Caucasian

Glutathione Coenzyme Q10 Flavonoids. By scavenging free radicals, these nutrients lower the chance of developing chronic illnesses.

Antioxidant-rich foods, including nuts, seeds, fruits, and vegetables, can help build a shield against the ravages of aging for the body and brain. Fatty Acids Omega-3 Omega-3 fatty acids' "anti-inflammatory and immune-modulating" qualities have made them powerful agents in the promotion of longevity. Among the sources of omega-3s are: Fish that is high in fat, such herring, mackerel, tuna, or salmon Flaxseeds Chia seeds Walnuts Plant oils, such as soybean and flaxseed oils. Fortified foods include soy milk, yogurt, juice, and cow's milk. A "risk factor associated with chronic inflammation" that is also linked to a number of age-related illnesses, such as cognitive loss, is growing older. Omega-3 fatty acids considerably improve cognitive function and aid to lessen the consequences of chronic inflammation.

Plant-Based Substances Plant-based chemicals, which are plentiful in fruits, vegetables, herbs, and spices, are super nutrients that offer a range of advantages for living a longer life. According to studies, "replacing meat-based foods with plant-based products will provide many valuable compounds" for a diet that "can help in the prevention of many diseases in addition to providing the necessary nutrients. Including a wide variety of plant-based foods in your diet will help you maximize the benefits of nature's longevity-promoting substances, such as: Fruits, Vegetables, Complete grains, Nuts, Seeds, Beans. Vegetables Polyphenols, for example, are plant-based chemicals that have been linked to better cellular function and a lower risk of disease.

Enhancing Diet to Promote Brain Health

Similar to how a well-maintained vehicle needs premium fuel to run at its best, your brain needs a certain nutritional pattern to function at its best cognitively. Your nutrition affects your brain health in more ways than just quelling hunger or controlling your weight. It helps support cognitive functions such as memory, focus, and attention. Here we have it:

Brain foods: foods that can help maximize mental function. Boosting Brain Function to Prevent Cognitive Decline Over time, these nutrients support the maintenance of your mental and cognitive capacities in addition to serving as strong protectors against the indicators of cognitive decline.

The B-vitamin family, which includes cobalamin (B12), pyridoxine (B6), and thiamine (B1), "is key players" in promoting the production of neurotransmitters.

Cognitive function, mood, and memory are significantly impacted by neurotransmitters, which are chemical messengers that let nerve cells communicate with one another. Among the nutritious foods rich in B-vitamins are the following: Lentils with Black Beans Eggs Yogurt with milk Clams, mussels, and oysters Chicken, Beef, and Pork Trout and Salmon Spinach Vital Minerals: Magnesium, Zinc, and Other Elements Numerous minerals are "reported to be protective against cognitive decline," and they all play important, diverse functions in maintaining brain health. These include magnesium, potassium, calcium, and zinc. These nutrients support structural integrity, modulate brain activity, strengthen memory, and facilitate signal transmission throughout the body and brain. Several instances of nutritious foods rich in vital minerals are as follows: Avocados Berries Watercress with Broccoli Cocoa Nuts and seeds from pumpkins Passion fruit with pineapple Delicious Potatoes Cheese and Yogurt

How the Brain and the Gut Are Related

The gut-brain axis, which is a connection between the two organs, was discovered, and this discovery caused a shift in our understanding of cognitive health. It highlights how the health of the gut has a substantial impact on mental health and calls attention to the connection that exists between the activity of the brain and the gastrointestinal tract. The gut-brain axis is a dynamic, "bidirectional communication network" that connects the enteric neural system of the gut to the central nervous system of the brain. This connection has been observed to exist between the two systems. The continuous flow of information that occurs through this connection has an effect on both the digestive system and the brain at the same time. Disturbances in this axis have been linked to emotional, neurological, and cognitive decline, according to a study.

What role does the microbiota in the gut play in brain function?

A diverse collection of bacteria that reside in the digestive system is known as the gut microbiota. This microbiota plays an essential role in the regulation of brain function. At the end of the day, they are "important for brain functions" that control mental activity and general well-being. The illness known as dysbiosis, which leads to an unbalanced community, has the potential to induce mental health problems such as anxiety, depression, and cognitive loss. One of the most important factors in reaching this balance and warding off certain diseases is consuming a diet that places an emphasis on nutrition and promotes lifespan. Maintaining a healthy gut flora also contributes to the body's reduction of inflammation, which boosts brain function. Reduced brain health is connected to neuroinflammation, "a potential mediator of cognitive impairments. Maintaining a well-balanced gut microbiota is an excellent way to promote both your current and long-term health. Shifting needs for a healthy body and mind accompany the internal and external changes that follow aging. Later in life, appetite changes frequently occur as a result of a general drop in hunger cues, changes in calorie requirements, or alterations in meal preferences. Dietary recommendations are also prone to change because research indicates that "older adults are at a greater risk of chronic diseases," which include heart disease, cancer, cognitive decline, loss of muscle mass, and osteoporosis. Nutrient shortages may emerge from this in conjunction with other age-related changes in metabolism and the body's capacity to absorb nutrients. Thankfully, these risks can be decreased with a balanced diet. Changing Nutrition and Diet for Aging People Adapting to the changes and making alterations to satisfy your nutritional needs is part of addressing the demands of aging.

Here are some dietary modifications you may make to encourage aging in a healthy manner:

Complete Protein: Protein is crucial for preserving muscle mass and improving health, and it "plays an important role in the health of older adults. To guarantee sufficient consumption, add lean protein sources like fish, chicken, beans, and lentils to meals and snacks. Protein-rich breakfasts and snacks can be produced by combining Greek yogurt, fruits, spinach, and a scoop of protein powder.

Increase your fiber consumption: Fiber helps you maintain healthy gut bacteria, aids digestion, and manages your weight. It's even "been demonstrated to lower bodily inflammation. Good reassets of fiber consist of fruits, vegetables, legumes, and complete grains. Increase your dietary fiber intake by ingesting fiber-rich snacks such as nuts, seeds, and dried fruits.

Maintain Hydration: Age-related increases in the risk of dehydration are "caused by changes in water and sodium balance and a lack of thirst sensation. The demands for hydration also alter with age. Use smartphone programs or alarms to remind yourself to drink water to stay hydrated. Additionally, you can add things high in water content to your diet, like fruits, vegetables, and low-sodium soups.

Include fasting: time-restricted food, sometimes known as intermittent fasting, can help regulate weight and promote metabolic health when done properly. Studies suggest that interval fasting is "accompanied by positive effects on cardiovascular disease, diabetes, autoimmunity, cancer, neurodegeneration, and aging risk factors. In order to achieve these advantages, some kinds of intermittent fasting combine intervals of eating and fasting. The majority of humans prefer longer lives. However, living a longer life also involves having a better quality of life, involving improved mental and physical health as well as the ability for independence and activities. As a registered dietitian, I have seen numerous people who are healthier than people half their age who are in their 70s, 80s, and beyond. Nutrition plays a big part in the riddle, but lifestyle factors are more essential than genes. According to research referenced in a 2016 review of the literature published in the journal Immunity & Aging, lifestyle variables influence longevity to the tune of 25%.

Here are five dietary behaviors you can take to boost your chances of living a longer life and savoring each year to the fullest.

Consume fruits and veggies. Eating more produce is, in my opinion, one of the most significant and beneficial habits you can establish. I recognize you pay attention this one a lot. Regretfully, the majority of Americans are spectacularly inaccurate. About one in ten adults in the United States does not consume enough fruits and vegetables, according to the Centers for Disease Control and Prevention (CDC). Merely 10% of individuals achieve the daily requirement of two to three cups of veggies, and 12% accomplish the daily target of one and a half to two cups of fruit. Aside from improving your vitamin consumption, attaining those minimums could prolong your life. A 2017 meta-analysis that was presented in the International Journal of Epidemiology revealed that eating more fruits and vegetables is connected to a decreased likelihood of dying from any cause, including cancer and heart disease. Try to get in five or more servings each day. More is OK, but according to multiple studies, there is no further risk of death at this limit.

How to Consume More Vegetables and Fruits Every day, aim to include two cups of fruit and three cups of vegetables (one cup is roughly the size of a tennis ball). Several pointers Make it a habit to have a cup of fruit for breakfast every day and another cup as part of your daily snack. Add one cup of vegetables to your lunch and two to your dinner. can mix and combine them. Two points are awarded for a smoothie consisting of a cup of frozen berries and a handful of greens. Additionally, you may include fresh fruit in stir-fry recipes and entrée salads by slicing apples or oranges.

Consume more Nuts. Nuts are a powerhouse of nutrients. They include vital nutrients including potassium and magnesium, fiber, antioxidants, plant protein, and healthy fats and vitamins.

It makes sense that they are tied to prolonging life. The metabolic syndrome, also known as insulin resistance syndrome, is a combination of illnesses that raise a person's risk of heart disease, diabetes, and stroke, according to the National Heart, Lung, and Blood Institute (NHLBI). The Journal of Nutrition published a larger study in 2020 that included a randomized trial that tracked 5,800 men and women with metabolic syndrome for a full year. The data indicate that various indicators related to metabolic syndrome declined with increased nut consumption. These indicators include weight, BMI, systolic blood pressure, waist circumference, and cholesterol levels. The study's female participants exhibited an increase in HDL, or good cholesterol, but not in the male individuals.

How to Consume More Nuts; Two tablespoons of nut butter also qualify as a serving; however, an ounce of nuts is nearly equal to a quarter cup. Nut butter can be used as a dip for fresh fruit or celery, mixed into smoothies, or stirred into cereal. Nuts can be eaten raw or added to stir-fry dishes, sautéed veggies, and salads. When coating fish or adding a garnish to dishes like mashed cauliflower or lentil soup, crushed almonds work brilliantly as a substitute for bread crumbs. Another fantastic technique to enhance your consumption is to bake with nut flours or use them in pancakes.

Consume more meatless foods. Mondays have been a thing for years. That's excellent, but for longevity, you should add plant-based meals to your eating regimen more than once a week. In a 2016 paper withinside the American Journal of Lifestyle Medicine, researchers define 5 areas withinside the global wherein human beings stay the longest, healthiest lives. Deemed Blue Zones, these places are located in widely various areas, from Okinawa, Japan, to Ikaria, Greece. One characteristic they share is the intake of mostly plant-based foods. Beans and lentils are cornerstones, and meat is eaten on average approximately five times per month in three- to four-ounce portions—roughly the size of a deck of cards. The sole Blue Zone in the US is in Loma Linda, California, which has the biggest population of Seventh-day Adventists. This group, noted for their predominantly plant-based diet, lives, on average, 10 years longer than their North American counterparts.For example, a 2013 study published in JAMA Internal Medicine looked at over 73,000 Seventh-day Adventist men and women and showed that, compared to omnivores, those who remained on a vegetarian diet had a considerably decreased overall mortality risk. This comprised vegans, lacto-ovo vegetarians (who do consume dairy and eggs), and pesco-vegetarians (who do eat shellfish). A 2019 follow-up study to the 2013 one, published in the Journal of Nutritional Science, indicated that, compared to the diet of nonvegetarians, vegetarian diets were associated with significantly reduced levels of cardiovascular disease risk factors. And in a 2022 take a look at in PLOS Medicine, researchers tested how meals alternatives have an effect on lifestyles expectancy. They discovered that the highest benefits to longevity may be gained by "eating more legumes, whole grains, and nuts, and less red and processed meat.

How to Eat Less Meat To gain the advantages; switch the meat in meals for pulses, the umbrella name for beans, lentils, peas, and chickpeas. Opt for lentil or black bean soup at the facet in preference to including fowl to a salad. Use black-eyed peas in a stir-fry in place of meat, and nibble on veggies with hummus instead of jerky. Explore ethnic eating places on your community that provide pulse-primarily based totally cuisine, like Indian chickpea curry and Ethiopian lentil stew.

Eat like a Mediterranean. When it comes to lifespan, it's the total eating pattern, rather than one meal or dietary group, that's crucial. A Mediterranean weight-reduction plan stays one of the gold requirements for dwelling longer and greater healthfully. This pattern is characterized by a large intake of fruits and vegetables; whole grains; pulses; nutritious fats from nuts, olive oil, and avocado; and herbs and spices. It contains seafood a couple times a week. The Mediterranean diet also involves moderate consumption of dairy, eggs, and wine and limits the intake of meat and sweets. One indicator of longevity often cited in studies at the cellular level is telomere length. In a nutshell, telomeres are caps found at the ends of chromosomes that safeguard DNA. When they end up too short, a mobileular will become antique or dysfunctional. This is why shorter telomeres are connected with a decreased life expectancy and an increased chance of developing chronic diseases. Research published in 2017 in the journal Oncotarget reveals that higher adherence to a Mediterranean diet is connected to longevity through maintaining longer telomere length. The same study indicated that for each one-point increment in the Mediterranean diet score (which evaluates adherence to the diet), the risk of dying from any cause lowers by 4 to 7%.

How to Eat a Mediterranean Diet; To Mediterraneanize your meals, substitute butter with nut butter or avocado on toast and trade it for extra virgin olive oil to sauté vegetables. Snack on fresh fruit with almonds, olives, or roasted chickpeas, and keep meals simple. A balanced Med-diet supper may consist of fish served over a bed of greens tossed in extra virgin olive oil with a side of roasted potatoes or quinoa and a glass of pinot noir.

Sip green tea. I like to refer to green tea as preventative medication in a mug. Numerous studies have connected it to a lower risk of heart disease, cancer, type 2 diabetes, Alzheimer's, and obesity. In a 2022 review of the literature published in the journal Nutrients, researchers discovered that people with the highest green tea intake had reduced rates of cardiovascular disease as nicely as a decrease threat of demise from coronary heart disorder and stroke. And while it cannot be said definitively that drinking green tea will make you live longer, there does seem to be some correlation between lifespan and green tea intake.

How to Drink More Green Tea In addition to sipping; you can use green tea as the liquid in smoothies, porridge, overnight oats, or to steam veggies or whole grain rice. It can also be included in soups, stews, sauces, and marinades. Matcha, a powdered version of green tea, can also be utilized in beverages and recipes. Just be sure to cut out any coffee at least six hours before bedtime so you won't impair your sleep length or quality.

A Quick Review: As far as what not to do, it's the typical suspect. Don't overeat or consume too much sugar, processed meals, meat, or alcohol. The good news is that the preventive foods listed can simply supplant aging-inducing diets. Reach for an apple with nut butter in place of processed cookies, and replace soda with green tea. In other words, focus on what to consume, and you'll naturally curb your intake of foods to avoid. That's significant because, for lifespan, consistency is key. A long-haul diet encourages a long, healthy life!

CHAPTER FOUR

TOP ANTI-AGING FOODS TO FIT INTO YOUR DIET

These anti-aging foods can help you eat your way to a longer life expectancy. Add these delectable items to your everyday diet, and you will be minimizing your risk for illnesses and age-related disorders. Just pick one or two to add to each week.

AVOCADOS:

Avocados have to be one of the most delectable meals out there. Mix up a little guacamole or slice a couple up on your salad for an anti-aging treat. Avocados are one of the best foods around for anti-aging and longevity. First of all, they are wonderful. But more significantly, avocados are rich with healthy fats and other nutrients to help your body live longer and operate better.

WALNUTS:

Walnuts are the best snack for anti-aging. They give you protein and omega-3s in a safe, easy way. Eat a handful of them every day. Walnuts are a wonderful anti-aging food because of the amount of omega-3s in just a handful. These omega-3 fatty acids are real lifespan tools. They fend off heart disease by boosting your HDL cholesterol level. Make walnuts part of your day, every day.

VEGETABLES:

Eating your vegetables for anti-aging may not seem like exciting advice, but the influence of eating enough vegetables on your life expectancy is extreme. Vegetables are an brilliant supply of vitamins and antioxidants. Not most effective that, however greens additionally assist you lose weight. Eat five to nine servings per day to help your body make repairs and live longer.

WATER:

Our bodies need water to fend off aging and damage. Drink lots of water every day to keep your body functioning efficiently. Water is a multi-billion-dollar industry. There are various claims that drinking water may "detox" your body. Most of these statements are not fully backed by research. However, drinking sufficient water is vital for numerous reasons, including getting rid of waste. And drinking water is a healthier alternative than sugary beverages full of empty calories.

CHOCOLATE: The fact that chocolate has anti-aging qualities is proof that the cosmos is a kind and caring place. Eat chocolate (now no longer too much) for anti-growing old benefits. Chocolate is one of the world's favorite foods. Recent research reveals that eating reasonable amounts of dark chocolate also delivers health benefits to the heart. The antioxidants in darkish chocolate defend your coronary heart towards aging, damage, and coronary heart disease.

BERRIES:

For an anti-aging dessert, try a bowl full of berries. Pack on those vitamins and avoid sugary substitutes. Berries are a rich source of antioxidants and other minerals. Eat extra strawberries, blueberries, and blackberries to assist with anti-getting older and longevity. Not only do berries battle free radicals that cause damage to your body, but they also contain other critical minerals. Work berries into your weekly diet.

RED WINE:

Good news! Red wine contains qualities that make you younger. Just a glass or two a day offers incredible anti-aging properties. Red wine is believed to provide a range of health benefits. Numerous scientific studies show the benefits of red wine.

GREEN TEA:

Green tea is an ancient drink for excellent health and life. The antioxidant advantages of daily drinking green tea are widely recognized. A tiny drink of inexperienced tea more than one instances an afternoon should do wonders in your existence expectancy. Abe SK, Saito E, Sawada N, et al. Green tea consuming and mortality in Japanese guys and women: a pooled evaluation of 8 population-primarily based totally cohort research in Japan

MELONS:

Melons are tasty. They are also an excellent source of a wide spectrum of vitamins. Eat a different sort of melon every week for tremendous health benefits. Melons are a fantastic source of vitamins and other nutrients. Watermelons and cantaloupe are easy-to-discover and less expensive reassets of great anti-getting old foods. Add melons to your everyday foods for a great nutritional boost to your diet.

BEANS:

As a ways as anti-getting old meals go, beans are one of the exceptional around. Your heart will adore the healthful, fat-free protein and other anti-aging qualities of beans. Beans are a wonderful anti-aging and lifespan diet. They offer healthful protein with out all of the fats which you locate in animal products. Beans also provide a huge supply of antioxidants that protect against damage from free radicals. Work beans into your weekly menu for their anti-aging effects.

CHAPTER FIVE

LONGEVITY DRUG THAT CAN SLOW THE AGEING PROCESS

Researchers throughout the world are researching different strategies to alter the biology of aging, says Jamie Justice, PhD, researcher and assistant Professor of gerontology and geriatric medication at Wake Forest School of Medicine in Winston Salem, North Carolina. "Many one of a kind capability interventions had been used on animal fashions which can boom how lengthy someone or organism lives, known as lifespan, and the way nicely they stay inside those years, called 'healthspan,'" adds Dr. Justice. Metformin has some properties that make it stand out among the many drugs being examined, she says. "While a number of those capsules haven't been researched or used a lot or have aspect results which can be probably risky, metformin has been used considerably for many years and has a good safety profile. The most prevalent side effects are GI disorders such as nausea and diarrhea," says Justice. And while some medications appear to target aging or disease via a single mechanism, metformin appears to positively impact numerous important pathways, says Justice. "Studies have already proven that metformin can put off growing older and enhance fitness in animals, and it can additionally impact essential growing older elements that underlie a couple of age-associated situations in humans," she says. "Metformin's widespread effects on metabolic and cellular processes, coupled with its well-established safety profile and low cost, make it an ideal candidate drug to extend a healthy lifespan in older adults," adds Justice.

Metformin isn't the only medicine with anti-aging promise. Another is rapamycin, a medicine intended to prevent transplant patients from rejecting donated organs. What sets metformin apart is the fact that it's a widely available generic medicine that is quite safe, Justice explains. Right now, most of the evidence about metformin's impact on longevity comes from research involving mice and worms. But the results of these animal experiments have been limited and usually only meaningful when metformin is begun at a young age. "When researchers have checked out metformin use in mice, it hasn't had profound consequences on how lengthy they live, however studies does advise that taking metformin can expand the healthspan of mice and other organisms," adds Justice. That may be important to the research on health span and lifespan in people, she says. A meta-evaluation posted in October 2022 in Aging Cell, Justice says, located that even as metformin wasn't drastically related to prolonging lifespan for mice or worms, the mice did display upgrades in insulin resistance and decrease degrees of oxidative stress, which performs a key function in lots of continual diseases. Lower ranges of oxidative pressure permit cells to restore any harm extra effectively. "Overall, the mice taking metformin seemed healthier. They walked around more and better; their fur looked a little nicer, and this has been repeated in a few studies," Justice says. For people with diabetes, metformin lowers the risk of death. Research in humans reveals that metformin can affect mortality. A meta-analysis published in 2017 that included 53 separate trials indicated that metformin reduces all-cause mortality and diseases of aging, independent of its effect on diabetes. The investigation indicated that the use of metformin reduced the risk of cancer, cardiovascular disease, stroke, and mortality, says Justice. "The findings on mortality risk are remarkable. People with diabetes on metformin have a lower risk of death than both those with diabetes who are not taking metformin or taking other drugs (such as sulphonylureas or insulin) and those without diabetes," she says. Diabetes is regarded as "accelerate" aging, meaning people with diabetes have a greater risk of developing another chronic disease and a greater risk of dying, according to Justice. "That someone taking metformin with diabetes may moreover have a lower danger of loss of life than someone without diabetes is truely promising for functionality results on human lifespan. But this needs to be validated definitively in a randomized clinical study, not merely epidemiology or medical records," she says. Researchers have recognised for a while that metformin does greater than simply help in reducing blood sugar, says Chris Triggle, PhD, a researcher and professor of pharmacology at Weill Cornell Medicine in Doha, Qatar. "The use of metformin has been shown to reduce the risk of and mortality associated with cardiovascular disease," he explains. There's also indication that it could aid in reducing age-related cognitive deterioration, according to a study published in January 2021 in Aging Cell. Metformin can result in moderate weight loss. On average, most people lose roughly six pounds after being on metformin for a year, according to a study. This small weight loss is "an obvious benefit for many people with type 2 diabetes," Dr. Triggle says, which "thereby could enhance healthspan and lifespan." "But it's important to note that metformin isn't really a weight loss drug, and most people don't lose a significant amount of weight from taking it," says Ashok Shetty, PhD, a researcher, professor, and associate director at the Institute for Regenerative Medicine at Texas A&M Medicine in Bryan, Texas. Though dropping even a tiny quantity of weight should assist enhance or maybe save you a few persistent diseases, researchers are capable of rent statistical methods to "tease out" the effects of weight loss, according to Justice. "Even after weight is managed for, studies indicates that there are still [health] advantages and upgrades to taking metformin," she says. Can metformin help people who don't have diabetes? In the Diabetes Prevention Program research, people without diabetes were offered exercise, metformin, or a placebo to delay diabetes. At the end of the study, metformin appeared to cut the incidence of diabetes by 30 percent. "Because of that, metformin is permitted for human beings who've pre-scientific diabetes," stated Nir Barzilai, MD, director of the Institute for Aging Research at Albert Einstein College of Medicine withinside the Bronx, New York, in an interview in Lifespan.io, an employer devoted to elevating price range to analyze growing old and age-associated diseases. Many people who don't have diabetes nonetheless get metformin, Dr. Barzilai pointed out. The difficulty is the absence of studies to back it up. "There are fewer research approximately individuals who are completely normal—llean and healthy," he said.

How does metformin affect the body?

Research has connected the positive effects of metformin to its activation of the enzyme AMPK (AMP-activated protein kinase), which plays numerous critical functions in the control of cell metabolism, adds Triggle. AMPK has been called the "gasoline gauge of the cell" due to the fact studies suggests it regulates power stability and different drivers of getting older and lifespan, which includes metabolism, resistance To stress, mobileular survival and growth, and autophagy, that is the body's method of reusing antique and broken mobileular parts. In addition to metformin, calorie restriction has been shown to activate AMPK, which has also been related to improving lifespan in multiple experimental trials, says Triggle. More studies is wanted to verify metformin's anti-getting old benefits. Based on the data that is now available, it's very difficult to distinguish the favorable effects of metformin in lowering type 2 diabetes from all the other health benefits, including anti-aging, according to Triggle. Triggle was the principal author of a manuscript published in August 2022 in the journal Metabolism that consolidated all the known data on metformin. His team concluded that "the evidence that metformin increases lifespan remains controversial" and that more data from "appropriately designed clinical trials is required."

Trials to Evaluate Metformin's Anti-Aging Effects Are in the Works Fundraising for the Targeting Aging with Metformin (TAME) experiment is now underway. The study intends to find out whether patients using metformin will have delayed development or progression of age-related chronic diseases such as heart disease, cancer, and dementia. The six-year research seeks to include roughly 3,000 participants between the ages of 65 and 79 years old. Researchers are striving to discover biomarkers that can measure the aging process and show if metformin is functioning or not. Without established biomarkers, it may take decades to undertake a randomized trial to prove if a medicine safely increases life. Investigators hope that the participants on metformin will have a delay in major age-related events and associated favorable changes in biomarkers of aging. Because metformin is so affordable—just a penny a tablet, according to Justice—there isn't much desire or incentive for drug companies to support the research, adds Justice, who serves as a member of the trial committee for TAME. It's also been tough because the research is "outside the box," in that it isn't looking at one specific disease but rather the overall aging process. If proven effective as an anti-aging drug, metformin could have a big impact. Even though metformin's status as an ultra-cheap generic has made trial fundraising difficult, it could be highly useful later if the drug is proved to have positive effects, says Justice. "We don't need to pop out with a drug to boom lifespan and fitness that only a few human beings can have enough money to take and could widen disparities," she says. If proved to be successful, the low price and availability of metformin advise it'd have a population-huge effect, provides Justice. Is it secure for folks that don't have diabetes to take metformin? Is it appropriate to use metformin to try to live longer, even if you don't have diabetes? That relies upon on who you speak to, aleven though professionals agree that earlier than taking metformin (or any prescription drug, for that matter), you must speak together along with your doctor. Unless you're taking part in a medical study, it might now no longer be recommended to apply metformin besides to deal with kind 2 diabetes or polycystic ovarian syndrome (PCOS), provides Triggle, despite metformin being a typically well-tolerated and safe medicine. "For instance, metformin isn't always utilized in sufferers with seriously decreased renal function. It is always good to seek and acquire counsel from a health expert before taking any medication," he says. Besides, metformin is not an over-the-counter nutritional supplement; you need a prescription from a doctor, according to Dr. Shetty. "You should only take this under a doctor's supervision. Lower dosages of metformin are quite safe," he says, although in rare cases, higher doses can contribute to a condition called lactic acidosis. "That's while lactic acid builds up withinside the bloodstream, that is a scientific emergency and might also be fatal," he says. Because metformin's purported benefits come from lowering oxidative stress and inflammation, it may not provide much benefit for younger people, according to Shetty. "Typically, the benefits would be better for middle-aged and older individuals," he explains. The Bottom Line on Metformin as an Anti-Aging Drug "There are dangers that include taking any drug, and that consists of metformin," explains Justice. Although there are incidents of doctors prescribing it off-label, for now most doctors are waiting for more proof—ssuch as the sort TAME may provide—bbefore recommending this to patients, she says. Can You Lengthen Your Life? Want the name of the game to residing an extended and more healthy life? Scientists have developed techniques to prolong the healthy lifespans of worms, mice, and even monkeys. Their work has offered interesting new insights regarding the biology of aging. But reliable data still shows that the greatest strategy to enhance the possibility of living a long and active life is to follow the advice you presumably received from your parents: eat well, exercise often, get plenty of sleep, and keep away from bad habits. People born in the U.S. nowadays can anticipate to stay to a median age of approximately 79. A century ago, lifestyles expectancy became in the direction of 54. "We've had a substantial boom in lifespan over the past century," says Dr. Marie Bernard, deputy director of NIH's National Institute on Aging. "Now in case you make it to age 65, the probability that you'll make it to eighty five may be very high. And if you make it to 85, the likelihood that you'll make it to 92 is pretty strong. So humans are residing longer, and it's occurring throughout the globe." Older parents have a tendency to be more healthy nowadays, too. Research has shown that healthy activities can help you stay active and healthy into your 60s, 70s, and beyond. In fact, a long-time period have a look at of Seventh-day Adventists—a spiritual company with a normally wholesome lifestyle—indicates that they generally tend to stay more healthy into antique age. Their life expectancy is roughly 10 years longer on average than that of most Americans. The Adventists' age-enhancing activities include frequent exercise, a vegetarian diet, avoiding tobacco and alcohol, and keeping a healthy weight. "If I needed to rank behaviors in phrases of priority, I'd say that workout is the maximum crucial issue related to residing longer and healthier," says Dr. Luigi Ferrucci, an NIH geriatrician who oversees studies on aging and health. "Exercise is especially important for lengthening active life expectancy, which is life without disease and without physical, mental, or cognitive disability." Natural changes to the body as we age can contribute to a progressive loss of muscle, less energy, and achy joints. These changes may make it appealing to move less and sit more. But doing that can enhance your risk for disease, disability, and even death. It's crucial to work with a doctor to determine the types of physical activities that can help you retain your health and mobility.

Even feeble older folks can benefit from frequent physical activity. One NIH-funded study included nearly 600 seniors, ages 70 to 89, who were at risk for impairment. They were randomly allocated to either a moderate exercise program or a comparator group without scheduled exercise. The exercise group steadily built up to 150 minutes of weekly activity. This includes vigorous walking, strength-and-balance training, and flexibility exercises. "After extra than 2 years, the bodily hobby institution had much less disability, and in the event that they have become disabled, they had been disabled for a shorter time than the ones withinside the comparison group," Bernard continues. "The mixture of diverse varieties of exercise—aerobic, strength and balance training, and flexibility—is critical to healthy aging." NIH's Go4Life net webweb page includes recommendations to help older human beings start and live active. Another definite way to increase your chances of a longer, healthier life is to lose extra weight. "Being obese—with a body mass index (BMI) higher than 30—is a risk factor for early death, and it shortens your active life expectancy," Ferrucci explains. BMI is an estimation of your body fat based on your weight and height. Use NIH's BMI calculator to estimate your BMI. Talk with a doctor about obtaining a healthy weight. Studies in animals have indicated that certain sorts of dietary changes—such as extremely low-calorie diets—can lead to longer, healthier lives. These studies offer information on the biological processes that affect healthy aging. But to date, calorie-restricted diets and other dietary adjustments have had mixed outcomes in extending the healthy lives of people.

CONCLUSIONS

The United States of America has had a slower rate of life expectancy growth during the previous quarter of a century compared to the advancements that have been made in a great number of other high-income countries. The United States of America has been continuously decreasing in the international rankings for level of life expectancy, and the gap between the United States and countries with the greatest achieved life expectancies has been expanding. This is a consequence of the fact that the United States has been declining consistently. Life expectancy at birth in the United States for both sexes combined presently ranks 28th in the world, slightly behind the United Kingdom, Korea, and Malta and more than 2 years in the back of Australia, Canada, France, Iceland, Italy, Japan, and Switzerland (United Nations, 2009). When compared to other countries, the United States of America exhibits comparable patterns of disadvantage when it comes to a variety of self-reported health metrics and biological markers of disease.

The patterns of mortality in older age groups can be found at: It is hardly surprising that disparities in levels of life expectancy exist among diverse high-income countries. It is probably more unexpected that major differences did not exist across many nations with high incomes around the year 1950, that the divergence that is being examined in this report started quite quickly around the year 1980, and that it has taken such a long time for this divergence to be discovered and analyzed. The divergence has happened for both men and women, as well as for ages above and below 50, when one examines trends in life expectancy at various ages across countries. This becomes apparent when one considers the fact that the divergence has occurred. According to the findings of this paper, the most significant disparity between countries appears to have been observed in the case of women aged 50 and older. This particular demographic has been the primary focus of the investigation. In the field of demography, descriptive analysis can be an extremely useful technique. In this case, the panel performed a comprehensive study of cause-of-death statistics to see whether certain causes of death could account for the comparatively low level of life expectancy in the United States and were connected with gains in life expectancy in leading countries. Comparative analysis of causes of death is hampered by issues of heterogeneity in coding procedures across nations and throughout time. Nevertheless, it does appear that higher mortality rates for lung cancer and respiratory disorders in the United States, Denmark, and the Netherlands are a significant part of the story. Such a finding is certainly consistent with the notion that smoking was a significant factor accounting for the slowdown of mortality decline among women in these three nations.

Other problems that account for the poor performance of U.S. women include cerebrovascular ailments (mainly stroke), diabetes, and mental disorders. Stroke is any other purpose of loss of life for which smoking is a hazard factor. Obesity is a danger issue for each stroke and diabetes. With respect to mental problems, the increase in such disorders is difficult to interpret, and the suggestion that this increase is linked to changes in coding cannot be rejected. It should be emphasized, however, that the risk factors for heart disease, diabetes, and stroke overlap with those for Alzheimer's disease, and it is probable that the trend in fatalities due to mental diseases is attributable to some of the same underlying reasons. Although mortality from coronary heart sickness performed little function withinside the divergent traits in existence expectancy—due to the fact even 50 years in the past the USA already had an awful lot better stages of mortality from heart disease than the other countries examined for this study—it accounts for about half the current gap between the United States and the countries with the highest life expectancies; Therefore, this circumstance must be a focal point of efforts to deliver U.S. life expectancy in line with that of the exemplar countries.

While a descriptive examination of causes of death is clearly informative, this paper has initiated the process of going from description to identifying the underlying determinants of the observed variations, a vital first step toward finally constructing an integrated model of causative processes. More precisely, the panel analyzed a variety of putative risk variables and considered how differences among nations in exposure to these risk factors would explain observed discrepancies in life expectancy. Such an approach is not without its drawbacks. For some factors, comparable cross-country statistics exist on the current levels of risk, while for others, shockingly little direct information can be brought to bear. Few countries are conducting systematic surveillance of health risk factors, so directly comparable data even for the present is often not available for a large number of countries, and For a sizeable wide variety of countries, information are to be had for nearly no danger elements for the 50-yr length tested for this study. Much is known about contemporary international differences in smoking behaviors and levels of obesity, but substantially less about international differences in stress, physical exercise, or social networks. 1 Furthermore, very little is known regarding changes over time and across countries in lifetime exposures and behaviors for most risk variables. The fluid nature of the association between mortality and some of the primary risk factors also hindered the panel's job. For example, the epidemiological literature still reveals large variations of opinion with respect to the size of the connection between obesity and mortality. As the obesity epidemic has grown, the number of people at risk of obesity-related health problems has climbed. At the same time, however, care for some of the more serious obesity-related health conditions, such as heart disease and type 2 diabetes, has improved. Thus, the net effect of increased obesity on mortality is difficult to measure.

Acknowledging those limitations, the panel's method become to try and set up the power of the proof for some of the maximum generally proffered factors for variations in existence expectancy among the US and different high-profits countries—for example, that those variations are the end result of a specifically inefficient U.S. fitness care device or that they're a feature of negative fitness behaviors withinside the United States, in particular with recognize to smoking, overeating, and failing to exercising sufficiently. The panel also addressed disparities among countries in degrees of social integration and in socioeconomic disparity. Ultimately, all of those capability danger elements will want to be tested in an incorporated framework throughout the whole lifestyles course, taking account of the results of variations in Socioeconomic status, behavioral chance factors, and social policy, in addition to results throughout unique cohorts and periods. Smoking appears to be responsible for a substantial part of the divergence in female life expectancy.

Other factors, like obesity, nutrition, exercise, and economic inequality, have likely played a part in explaining the current difference between the United States and other nations, but evidence of their contribution to the divergence is not as firm. The case against smoking, by comparison, is fairly solid. Fifty years ago, smoking was far more widespread in the United States than in Europe or Japan; a larger proportion of Americans smoked and smoked more intensively than was the situation in other nations. The health effects of this conduct are still playing out in today's mortality rates. Over the period 1950–2003, the gain in life expectancy at age 50 was 2.1 years shorter among U.S. women compared with the average of nine other high-income countries (5.7 vs. 7.8 years gained, respectively). The damage caused by smoking was projected to account for 78 percent of the discrepancy in life expectancy for women and 41 percent of the deficit for men between the United States and other high-income nations in 2003 (Chapter 5).

Smoking has also caused considerable reductions in life expectancy in the Netherlands and Denmark, which, as indicated, are two other countries with relatively poor life expectancy trends. It has had a big negative influence on life expectancy in Canada, where life expectancy trends have been much more positive. While smoking looks to be a major element of the plot, it is by no means the full story. Other factors, particularly the rising prevalence of obesity in the United States, also appear to have played a substantial influence, although, as indicated, there is a good deal of uncertainty in the research regarding the mortality effects of obesity and any trends therein. Several peer-reviewed publications coming recently imply effects of widely different orders of magnitude. Preston and Stokes (2010) find that, even with relatively low estimates of related risk, obesity accounts for a fifth to a third of the gap in life expectancy in the United States relative to other high-income nations. Other specific risk variables are also definitely essential, but their impacts are considerably more difficult to define. The panel discovered a few proof to signify that adults elderly 50 and over withinside the United States are really extra sedentary than the ones in Europe, however the studies base Is inadequate even to become aware of an inexpensive variety of uncertainty in estimates of the contribution of bodily pastime to worldwide variations or developments in mortality. In different circumstances, the panel judged that unique hazard elements are not likely to have performed a huge position withinside the divergence of lifestyles expectancy in diverse international locations over the past 25 years. A substantial amount of work suggests a causal association between social relationships, social integration, and mortality. Yet there is no justification for assuming that levels or trends in the quality of social networks have played a role in the various life expectancies analyzed. Similarly, no evidence supports the hypothesis that postmenopausal hormone therapy played a part in a developing longevity gap for American women. Finally, the panel considered whether disparities in health care systems between countries might help explain the divergence in life expectancy over the previous 25 years. The health care system in the United States differs from those in other high-income nations in a variety of areas that could possibly lead to disparities in life expectancy. Certainly, the absence of widespread access to health care in the United States has increased mortality and reduced life expectancy. However, that is a smaller aspect above age sixty five than at more youthful a while due to Medicare entitlements. For the leading causes of mortality at older ages—cancer and cardiovascular disease—available data do not suggest that the U.S. health care system is failing to prevent fatalities that would otherwise be averted. In reality, cancer detection and survival appear better in the United States than in most other high-income countries. Survival rates following a heart attack are likewise favorable in the United States. Most of the comparative statistics the panel analyzed pertain to the performance of the U.S. health care system relative to those of other high-income nations once an illness has already established itself. A further issue is that the U.S. health care system does a particularly bad job at prevention, a finding that may be especially important in the midst of a statewide obesity epidemic. The panel analyzed scattered material on the performance of the United States with respect to preventive medicine relative to European countries and concluded the evidence to be inconclusive. Certainly, the high frequency of some health disorders in the United States is consistent with a failure of preventative medicine. But it could also be compatible with a higher prevalence of smoking, obesity, and physical inactivity among Americans, or with a medical system that may be unusually adept at recognizing specific conditions.

There is little question that high mortality rates among persons of poor socio-economic class are one reason the United States has a lower level of life expectancy than it might otherwise. A useful indicator of socioeconomic position is educational level (Avendano et al., 2010). Death rates at certain levels of educational attainment tend to be greater in the United States than in other nations, and the discrepancies are often greatest at the lowest levels of education. On the other hand, lifetime socioeconomic position has generally been greater for these cohorts of Americans than for the corresponding cohorts of

Europeans. Because educational levels in the United States have been quite high, the low-education group is quite tiny in the United States, while the high-education group is quite large. As a result, measures of inequality in mortality that combine distributions with rates reveal that the United States is not uncommon in the size of its death differentials by educational level. Finding the impact of socioeconomic disparity in the divergence in life expectancy among high-income nations is more challenging than finding its involvement in mortality levels, although it appears to have played some influence. Data from the period after 1980 do imply, however, that growing inequality in mortality in the United States is linked to a halt in mortality improvement among white women, particularly those with low levels of education.

Finally, with respect to racial differentials, high mortality rates among blacks obviously help explain why the level of life expectancy in the United States is lower than it might otherwise be. However, racial inequalities in mortality are unlikely to add considerably to explanations for the variance in life expectancy between the United States and other high-income countries after 1980. Neither the relative size of the white and black populations nor the mortality differential between the two has altered substantially enough since that time for that differential to possess much explanatory power.

www.ingramcontent.com/pod-product-compliance
Lightning Source LLC
Chambersburg PA
CBHW050855260726
48660CB00006B/2648